THE

ENHANCED

ATHLETE

COOKBOOK

RECIPES FOR IMPROVED PERFORMANCE

FREE MEAL PLAN

Copyright © 2023 by Adam kabbani

TABLE OF CONTENTS

INTRODUCTION:

Welcome to The Enhanced Athlete Cookbook! This cookbook is designed to provide athletes of all levels with delicious, nutritious recipes and meal plans that will help optimize performance, aid in recovery, and support overall well-being. Whether you're a professional athlete, a weekend warrior, or someone who enjoys staying active, this cookbook will guide you on a culinary journey that perfectly complements your physical endeavors.

CHAPTER 1

POWER-PACKED BREAKFASTS

In the world of sports and athletics, breakfast is often considered the most essential meal of the day. Whether you are a professional athlete, an amateur sports enthusiast, or simply someone who leads an active lifestyle, a power-packed breakfast can make a world of difference in boosting your performance and overall well-being.

Power-packed breakfasts for athletes are specifically designed to provide the necessary nutrients, energy, and stamina required to excel in sporting activities. They are carefully crafted to optimize performance, enhance muscle recovery, and sustain energy levels throughout the day.

One of the key components of a power-packed breakfast is protein. Athletes need a sufficient amount of protein in their diet to aid in muscle growth and repair. Including protein-rich foods like eggs, Greek yogurt, lean meats, and plant-based options like tofu or lentils can provide the amino acids necessary for optimal muscle development.

Another vital element in an athlete's breakfast is carbohydrates. Carbohydrates serve as the primary source of energy for the body, especially during intense physical activity. Whole-grain cereals, oats, whole wheat bread, and fruits are excellent choices that provide a slow and steady release of energy for sustained performance.

Furthermore, healthy fats play a crucial role in supporting an athlete's cognitive function and overall health. Incorporating foods like avocados, nuts, and seeds can provide the necessary omega-3 fatty acids, which aid in brain function and reduce inflammation within the body.

Including a variety of vitamins and minerals in a power-packed breakfast can help optimize an athlete's overall health and well-being. Fruits and vegetables are excellent sources of antioxidants, vitamins, and minerals that support the immune system, aid in recovery, and reduce the risk of injury.

A power-packed breakfast is a combination of protein, carbohydrates, healthy fats, and essential vitamins and minerals. It fuels the body, enhances performance, and promotes optimal recovery. By incorporating these wholesome foods into their morning routine, athletes can set themselves up for success both on and off the field.

OATMEAL WITH FRUIT AND NUTS:

This power-packed breakfast is perfect for athletes as it combines complex carbohydrates from the oats, essential vitamins and minerals from the fruits, and healthy fats from the nuts. Oatmeal provides a sustained release of energy, while the fruits offer a variety of antioxidants to support recovery. Nuts, such as almonds or walnuts, are rich in protein and healthy fats, which aid in muscle repair and provide long-lasting energy.

Oatmeal with fruit and nuts is a delicious and nutritious breakfast dish that combines the heartiness of oats with the natural sweetness of fresh fruits and the added crunch of nuts. This dish is not only satisfying and easy to make, but it also provides a healthy start to your day.

Oatmeal serves as the base of this dish, providing a filling and nutritious grain. Oats are a great source of fiber, beta-glucan, vitamins, and minerals. They are known for lowering cholesterol levels, aiding digestion, and providing sustained energy. With their creamy texture and mild flavor, oats create a comforting and satisfying meal.

Adding fruits to your oatmeal not only enhances its taste but also provides a burst of vitamins and antioxidants. Fresh berries, such as strawberries, blueberries, or raspberries, are excellent choices as they are packed with vitamin C and other beneficial compounds. Their natural sweetness complements the oats perfectly, creating a delightful combination.

To further enhance the flavor, texture, and nutritional profile of your oatmeal, adding a variety of nuts is a great option. Almonds, walnuts, or pecans are all popular choices. These nuts offer a crunchiness that contrasts with the softness of the oats and adds a rich, nutty flavor. Nuts are also an excellent source of healthy fats, protein, and minerals, making this dish even more nutritious.

PROTEIN PANCAKES WITH GREEK YOGURT:

Protein pancakes made with ingredients like whole grain flour, eggs, and protein powder are a great choice for athletes. These pancakes provide a good balance of carbohydrates and protein, promoting muscle recovery and growth. Greek yogurt, when served as a topping, adds extra protein, calcium, and probiotics, which contribute to strong muscles and a healthy gut.

Protein Pancakes with Greek Yogurt are a delicious and nutritious breakfast option that is perfect for those looking to start their day with a protein-packed meal. These pancakes are not only tasty and satisfying, but they also provide the right amount of energy needed to kickstart your morning.

To make these pancakes, you'll need a combination of basic ingredients such as whole wheat flour, eggs, milk, and baking powder, along with a generous amount of Greek yogurt. Greek yogurt is a key ingredient in this recipe as it adds a creamy texture and rich flavor, while also providing a significant amount of protein. The addition of Greek yogurt not only enhances the taste and texture of the pancakes but also increases the nutritional value.

When cooked, these protein pancakes have a fluffy texture with a slightly tangy flavor from the Greek yogurt. They are incredibly versatile, allowing you to customize them to your liking. You can choose to add in your favorite fruits, such as blueberries or bananas, or sprinkle them with nuts or seeds for an added crunch. The possibilities are endless!

What makes these pancakes unique is the high protein content, which promotes muscle repair and growth. This is especially beneficial for those who follow a fitness regime or are looking to build lean muscle mass. Additionally, protein helps keep you feeling full for longer periods, which makes these pancakes an excellent option for weight management or as a pre or post-workout meal.

Overall, Protein Pancakes with Greek Yogurt are a tasty and wholesome way to start your day. Packed with protein, fiber, and essential nutrients, they not only satisfy your tastebuds but also provide a nutritious boost to keep you energized throughout the morning. So why not whip up a batch of these pancakes and experience the perfect fusion of deliciousness and health in one bite?

EGG AND VEGGIE SCRAMBLE WITH WHOLE WHEAT TOAST:

This breakfast option is packed with essential nutrients. Eggs are an excellent source of high-quality protein and provide essential amino acids required for muscle repair and growth. Adding a mix of chopped vegetables, such as spinach, bell peppers, and mushrooms, adds fiber, vitamins, and minerals. Serving it with whole wheat toast further boosts the intake of complex carbohydrates for sustained energy throughout the day.

Egg and Veggie Scramble with Whole Wheat Toast is a nutritious and delicious breakfast option that combines the goodness of eggs, a variety of colorful vegetables, and the heartiness of whole wheat toast. This flavorful dish is a perfect choice for those looking to start their day with a balanced meal.

The dish begins with a simple scramble of eggs, which are whisked until light and fluffy. The eggs are then cooked gently in a non-stick skillet until just set, creating a soft and creamy texture.

To make this scramble even more nutritious, a medley of fresh vegetables is added. Vibrant colors from chopped bell peppers, onions, and spinach not only enhance the visual appeal but also bring a burst of flavor and a range of important vitamins and minerals. The vegetables are sautéed until tender, resulting in a delightful combination of textures and tastes.

This egg and veggie scramble is perfectly complemented by a side of whole wheat toast. Whole wheat bread is a healthier alternative to refined white bread, as it is higher in fiber and nutrients. Toasted to perfection, the slices of whole wheat bread provide a satisfying crunch and serve as a delicious platform for the scramble.

The Egg and Veggie Scramble with Whole Wheat Toast is a versatile dish that can be customized to individual preferences. A sprinkle of cheese can be added for a creamy and slightly indulgent twist, while a dash of hot sauce or herbs can lend a bit of extra kick and aroma. It can be enjoyed as a quick weekday breakfast or as a leisurely weekend brunch option, providing a nourishing and filling start to the day.

An Egg and Veggie Scramble with Whole Wheat Toast provides numerous benefits to an athlete.

Eggs are an excellent source of high-quality protein, which is essential for muscle growth, repair, and recovery. The scramble also incorporates various vegetables, such as spinach, bell peppers, and tomatoes, which are rich in vitamins, minerals, and antioxidants. These nutrients support overall health, strengthen the immune system, and aid in preventing inflammation and oxidative stress.

Additionally, whole wheat toast provides complex carbs for sustained energy release, which is crucial for an athlete during training or competition. It also contains fiber, which promotes satiety and aids in digestion.

Overall, this nutritious meal helps athletes fuel their bodies, maintain optimal energy levels, support muscle development, and promote overall health and wellbeing.

HIGH-FIBER GRANOLA BARS

High-fiber granola bars are an essential addition to any athlete's diet as they provide a convenient and nutritious source of energy and essential nutrients. These bars are specifically designed to cater to the increased dietary needs of athletes, helping them perform at their best.

Packed with fiber, these granola bars offer numerous benefits to athletes. Fiber aids in digestion, promoting a healthy gut and preventing any discomfort during physical activities. It also helps regulate blood sugar levels, ensuring a steady release of energy during workouts or competitions. This sustained energy release is crucial for athletes, as it allows them to maintain optimal performance throughout their activities.

High-fiber granola bars are also rich in complex

carbohydrates, which are the primary source of fuel for athletes. These carbs are necessary to replenish glycogen stores in muscles, which can become depleted during intense training sessions or long-duration activities. By consuming these bars, athletes are able to efficiently refuel their bodies and feel energized for their next workout.

In addition to providing energy, high-fiber granola bars are often fortified with important vitamins and minerals. These include calcium, iron, and B vitamins, which are essential for maintaining strong bones, healthy blood cells, and optimal metabolism. These micronutrients are particularly crucial for athletes who place extra stress on their bodies, making these bars an excellent choice to support their overall health and athletic performance.

Furthermore, these granola bars are often made with natural and wholesome ingredients such as whole grains, nuts, seeds, and dried fruits. This ensures that athletes are fueling their bodies with real food nutrients rather than artificial additives or excess added sugars. The high-fiber content, combined with the natural ingredients, makes these bars a satiating snack that helps athletes feel full and satisfied for longer periods of time.

Overall, high-fiber granola bars are a must-have for any athlete looking to optimize their performance, maintain a healthy gut, and support their overall well-being. These bars offer a convenient and tasty solution to ensure athletes are properly fueled and nourished, no matter the intensity of their training or competition.

CHAPTER 2

WHOLESOME SNACKS

In today's health-conscious world, athletes strive to maintain optimal performance by focusing on not just their training regimen but also their nutrition. One aspect of an athlete's diet that significantly impacts their performance is snacking. Wholesome snacks play an integral role in an athlete's diet, providing them with the necessary nutrients, energy, and sustenance to fuel their bodies during training and competitions. This introduction will provide an overview of the importance of wholesome snacks for athletes, the key nutrients they should include, and examples of delicious and nutritious snack options.

Wholesome snacks are crucial for athletes as they provide a continuous supply of energy throughout the day. Athletes have high energy demands due to intense physical activity, and regular meals alone may not suffice to meet these requirements. Snacks can fill the gaps between meals, ensuring athletes have enough fuel to support their performance and recovery. Moreover, consuming wholesome snacks can help prevent hunger and cravings, leading to healthier food choices and avoiding overeating junk food.

When considering wholesome snacks for athletes, it is essential to include a balance of macronutrients and micronutrients. Carbohydrates are the primary source of energy for athletes and should be included in snacks to replenish glycogen stores. Protein is crucial for muscle repair and growth, making it important for post-workout snacks. Healthy fats provide sustained energy and aid in nutrient absorption. Additionally, snacking on foods rich in vitamins, minerals, and antioxidants helps support overall health and immune function.

Wholesome snacks play a vital role in an athlete's diet and can have a significant impact on their performance. By incorporating nutrient-dense snacks into their daily routine, athletes can ensure they are fueling their bodies with the necessary energy, macronutrients, and micronutrients. These snacks not only provide sustained energy but also support muscle repair, immune function, and overall health. With a wide variety of wholesome snack options available, athletes can enjoy delicious and nutritious choices that contribute to their success on and off the field.

GREEK YOGURT WITH BERRIES

This snack combines protein from Greek yogurt, which is also a great source of calcium, with antioxidant-rich berries for added vitamins and fiber.

Greek yogurt with berries is a delicious and nutritious treat that provides a powerhouse of energy and nutrients to fuel an athlete's active lifestyle. Made from strained yogurt, Greek yogurt is known for its thick and creamy texture, making it a satisfying and filling snack option.

Packed with protein, Greek yogurt is an excellent choice for athletes as it helps build and repair muscles before and after intense workouts. It contains twice the protein of regular yogurt, allowing athletes to meet their protein requirements without consuming excess calories. The protein in Greek yogurt also helps in maintaining a feeling of satiety, keeping hunger at bay and assisting with weight management.

Add to that the vibrant burst of color and incredible nutritional benefits of fresh berries, and you have a winning combination. Berries like blueberries, strawberries, raspberries, and blackberries are not only low in calories but also rich in vitamins, minerals, and antioxidants. These antioxidants help combat inflammation and oxidative stress caused by intense physical activity, reducing muscle soreness and enhancing recovery.

The natural sweetness of the berries adds a delightful flavor to the tangy Greek yogurt, making it an absolute pleasure to indulge in. Athletes can enjoy this treat as a snack in between meals, a post-workout recovery option, or even as a healthy dessert. Additionally, the carbohydrates from the berries provide a quick source of energy, replenishing glycogen stores to support endurance and performance.

You are a professional athlete or simply someone who leads an active lifestyle, Greek yogurt with berries is a delectable and nutritious option that meets all your dietary needs. So, grab a spoonful and enjoy the health benefits it has to offer.

Greek yoghurt with berries can be a game-changer for athletes. Firstly, it is a rich source of protein, which aids in muscle repair and recovery after intense workouts, helping athletes to bounce back quicker. The combination of Greek yoghurt and berries provides a good balance of carbohydrates and antioxidants, which can support energy levels and boost the immune system, keeping athletes healthy and resilient. The natural sugars found in berries also provide a quick source of energy, ideal for pre-workout fueling. Additionally, Greek yoghurt with berries is packed with vitamins and minerals, such as calcium, potassium, and vitamin C, which are essential for overall athletic performance and bone health.

NUT BUTTER WITH WHOLE-GRAIN BREAD

A perfect mix of healthy fats, protein, and complex carbohydrates, this snack provides sustained energy and essential nutrients for athletes.

As an athlete, you are constantly pushing your body to its limits, and fueling it with the right nutrients is crucial for optimal performance. One of the best and most wholesome options for a quick and healthy snack is nut butter with whole-grain breads.

Nut butter, such as almond or peanut butter, is an excellent source of healthy fats, protein, and essential vitamins and minerals. These healthy fats provide a slow and sustained release of energy, making it the perfect choice to boost your endurance during training sessions or competitions. Additionally, the high protein content helps repair and build muscles, supporting your athletic performance and recovery.

Pairing nut butter with whole-grain breads is a winning combination. Whole-grain breads are packed with complex carbohydrates, which are essential for providing your body with the energy it needs for intense workouts or competitions. These carbohydrates are digested more slowly than simple sugars, preventing energy crashes and ensuring a steady supply of fuel.

The combination of the healthy fats from nut butter and the complex carbohydrates from whole-grain breads creates a well-balanced snack that provides sustained energy throughout your workout or event. Unlike highly processed and sugary snacks, this wholesome option keeps your blood sugar levels stable, enhances focus and concentration, and helps you avoid the dreaded sugar crash.

Moreover, nut butter with whole-grain breads is incredibly versatile. You can mix it up by adding sliced bananas, berries, or a drizzle of honey for added flavor and extra nutrients. It's easy to prepare and can be packed in your gym bag or consumed as a pre or post-workout snack.

Nut butter with whole-grain breads is an excellent choice for athletes looking to fuel their bodies with nutrient-dense and energy-boosting snacks. It provides the perfect combination of healthy fats, protein, and complex carbohydrates to support your stamina, endurance, and overall athletic performance.

For athletes, incorporating nut butter with whole-grain breads into their diet offers numerous benefits. Firstly, nut butter serves as an excellent source of protein, which aids in muscle recovery and growth, supporting an athlete's training regime. The combination of nut butter and whole-grain bread provides a great balance of carbohydrates and healthy fats, supplying sustained energy during workouts and competitions. The natural oils present in nut butter contribute to joint health, reducing inflammation and supporting overall joint mobility, crucial for athletes' performance. Additionally, nut butter contains an array of vitamins and minerals, such as vitamin E, magnesium, and potassium, which are essential for overall health and immune function.

TRAIL MIX

A combination of nuts, dried fruits, and dark chocolate provides a balanced blend of carbohydrates, healthy fats, and antioxidants, making it an ideal on-the-go snack.

Trail mix is a versatile and nutrient-dense snack that is tremendously beneficial for athletes. It is a delicious combination of various nuts, dried fruit, seeds, and sometimes even chocolate or granola, making it both energizing and satisfying.

The nuts, such as almonds, walnuts, and cashews, provide a high amount of protein, healthy fats, and essential vitamins and minerals. These components are crucial for athletes, as they help in muscle recovery and growth, increase endurance, and support overall physical performance. The healthy fats found in nuts also aid in satiety and can help maintain a healthy weight.

Dried fruits, including raisins, cranberries, and apricots, offer a natural sweetness to trail mix while boosting its nutritional value. They are packed with antioxidants, vitamins, and fiber, which help in reducing inflammation, boosting the immune system, and aiding in digestion. The natural sugars found in dried fruits provide quick energy to athletes during intense workouts or competitions.

Seeds like sunflower or pumpkin seeds are often incorporated into trail mix to add a satisfying crunch. These tiny powerhouses are loaded with essential nutrients such as iron, magnesium, and omega-3 fatty acids. Iron promotes healthy blood circulation and oxygen transport, while magnesium contributes to muscle relaxation and can help prevent cramps. Omega-3 fatty acids are known for their anti-inflammatory properties and contribute to heart health.

Additionally, some varieties of trail mix may include dark chocolate or granola, which further enhance the taste and nutritional profile. The cacao in dark chocolate contains antioxidants that support cardiovascular health, and granola can offer a healthy dose of carbohydrates, fiber, and additional protein.

Overall, trail mix is a convenient and highly nutritious snack that provides a good balance of carbohydrates, proteins, and fats, making it an ideal choice for athletes. Consuming trail mix before or after exercise can replenish energy levels, provide key nutrients, and promote optimal physical performance.

VEGGIE STICKS WITH HUMMUS

Fresh vegetables such as carrots, cucumber, and bell peppers paired with protein-rich hummus make for a nutrient-dense snack that provides vitamins, minerals, and fiber.

As an athlete, you are well aware of the importance of maintaining a healthy and balanced diet to support your training and performance. One exceptional snack that perfectly complements your fitness routine is veggie sticks with hummus.

Veggie sticks are an ideal choice for athletes due to their high nutritional value and low-calorie content. These sticks are made from a variety of fresh vegetables, such as carrots, celery, bell peppers, and cucumber. Packed with essential vitamins, minerals, and dietary fiber, they provide a plethora of health benefits. For instance, their high vitamin A content supports healthy vision and boosts your immune system, while the potassium found in celery aids in maintaining proper muscle function and prevents cramping.

Pairing veggie sticks with hummus enhances their nutritional profile and adds a delicious flavor to the snack. Hummus is a Middle Eastern dip made primarily from chickpeas, olive oil, tahini, and garlic. The chickpeas supply a generous amount of plant-based protein, which is crucial for muscle recovery and growth. Additionally, the healthy fats derived from olive oil are known to promote heart health and reduce inflammation.

Together, veggie sticks and hummus offer athletes a winning combination. They provide a valuable source of energy, promote healthy digestion, and contribute to proper hydration. Moreover, they are quick, convenient, and easy to prepare, making them an excellent snack option to satisfy hunger cravings before or after workouts.

Veggie sticks with hummus serve as a nutritious and scrumptious choice for athletes like you, delivering a satisfying and wholesome snack that supports your training goals and enhances your overall well-being.

Veggie sticks with hummus provide numerous benefits to athletes. Firstly, they are rich in essential nutrients like vitamins, minerals, and antioxidants, which aid in optimal performance and recovery. The veggie sticks are packed with fiber, aiding digestion and promoting a healthy gut. This ensures athletes maintain a healthy body weight and have sustained energy levels throughout training and competitions.

Hummus, on the other hand, is a great source of plant-based protein, which is essential for repairing and building muscle tissues. It also contains healthy fats that help maintain joint health and reduce inflammation, which is crucial for athletes engaging in intense physical activities.

Moreover, this snack option is low in calories and contains no cholesterol or saturated fats, making it ideal for maintaining a balanced diet and promoting overall heart health. The combination of veggie sticks and hummus provides a delicious and convenient way for athletes to fuel their bodies with wholesome, nourishing ingredients.

PROTEIN SMOOTHIE

A smoothie made with a high-quality protein powder, fruits, vegetables, and a liquid of choice offers a nutritious and easily digestible snack option for athletes.

Protein smoothies can be a powerful addition to an athlete's diet. Packed with essential nutrients, here are some key benefits:

Protein smoothies have become an essential part of an athlete's diet and nutrition regimen. These delectable and nutritious beverages are specifically designed to support muscle recovery, enhance performance, and provide vital nutrients for optimal athletic functioning.

Packed with high-quality protein, typically derived from sources like whey, casein, or plant-based proteins such as soy or pea, protein smoothies are a practical and convenient way for athletes to meet their daily protein requirements. Protein is a crucial macronutrient required for muscle repair and growth, making it an invaluable component in an athlete's diet. Consuming protein smoothies after workouts or training sessions helps jumpstart the muscle repair process, reduce muscle soreness, and enhance muscle recovery.

In addition to protein, these smoothies contain an array of other nutrients, including carbohydrates, vitamins, and minerals. Carbohydrates help replenish glycogen stores, essential for prolonged endurance activities and optimal energy levels, while vitamins and minerals support overall health and aid in various metabolic processes.

Protein smoothies are often enriched with other sports nutrition ingredients, such as creatine, glutamine, or branched-chain amino acids (BCAAs). These additional supplements can further enhance recovery, reduce muscle damage, and promote muscle protein synthesis, leading to improved athletic performance.

Furthermore, protein smoothies offer a convenient and delicious way to consume nutrient-dense ingredients like fruits, vegetables, nuts, and seeds. By blending these ingredients together, athletes can easily incorporate a range of vitamins, minerals, and antioxidants into their diet to support overall health and wellbeing.

Whether enjoyed as a post-workout recovery drink, a meal replacement, or a healthy snack throughout the day, protein smoothies are a versatile and accessible option for athletes seeking optimal nutritional support. They provide a quick, delicious, and efficient way to meet their protein needs, refuel energy stores, and promote muscle recovery, ultimately helping athletes reach their performance and fitness goals.

these snacks deliver the necessary fuel for muscles, enabling athletes to perform at their best. Additionally, the balanced macronutrient composition of these snacks helps to maintain stable blood sugar levels, preventing energy crashes and promoting sustained performance.

Furthermore, wholesome snacks are rich in essential nutrients such as vitamins, minerals, and antioxidants. These nutrients play a vital role in supporting the immune system, reducing inflammation, and promoting overall health and well-being. By nourishing their bodies with wholesome snacks, athletes can optimize their recovery and minimize the risk of injuries and illnesses.

Moreover, wholesome snacks offer convenience and versatility, making them easily accessible for athletes on the go. Whether it's a homemade energy bar, a bag of mixed nuts, or a piece of fruit with nut butter, these snacks can be prepared and packed in advance, ensuring that athletes have a healthy option readily available whenever hunger strikes. This accessibility helps athletes make better choices and avoid reaching for unhealthy processed snacks or sugary alternatives.

Wholesome snacks serve as an integral part of an athlete's nutrition plan. They provide the necessary nutrients, energy, and convenience to support optimal performance and overall well-being. By incorporating these snacks into their diet, athletes can fuel their bodies, enhance their endurance, and promote recovery. Embracing wholesome snacks not only benefits athletes' athletic endeavors but also promotes long-term health and vitality. So, whether you're a professional athlete or a recreational enthusiast, consider the power of wholesome snacks to fuel your performance and achieve your athletic goals.

CHAPTER 3

PERFORMANCE-ENHANCING SALADS

The role of salads in enhancing athletic performance is often overlooked. However, with their combination of nutrient-dense ingredients, performance-enhancing salads have the potential to revolutionize the way athletes approach their diets and optimize their physical abilities.

Performance-enhancing salads are not your typical side dish; they are carefully crafted meals that pack a punch when it comes to nutritional value. These salads incorporate a wide variety of fresh vegetables, fruits, lean proteins, healthy fats, and complex carbohydrates to provide athletes with a well-rounded, nourishing meal that supports their training, performance, and recovery.

One of the primary benefits of performance-enhancing salads is their high nutrient density. The diverse array of colorful vegetables and fruits used in these salads offers a spectrum of vitamins, minerals, and antioxidants that are essential for optimal health and athletic performance. These nutrients play critical roles in energy metabolism, muscle function, immune support, and the prevention of oxidative stress. By consuming performance-enhancing salads, athletes can ensure that their bodies receive a wide range of nutrients necessary for peak performance.

Furthermore, performance-enhancing salads offer a balanced combination of macronutrients. They are typically designed to provide an optimal ratio of carbohydrates, proteins, and healthy fats to support athletic endeavors. Carbohydrates serve as the primary energy source, ensuring that athletes have the necessary fuel for intense training sessions and competitions. Proteins are vital for muscle repair and growth, aiding in recovery and optimizing performance. Healthy fats, such as those found in avocados or nuts, provide long-lasting energy, reduce inflammation, and support brain function. The synergy of these macronutrients in performance-enhancing salads ensures that athletes have a well-rounded, nourishing meal that supports their physical demands.

In addition to their nutrient density and macronutrient balance, performance-enhancing salads offer numerous other advantages for athletes. First, they are easily customizable, allowing athletes to tailor their salads to their specific dietary needs and preferences. Whether it's incorporating plant-based proteins, whole grains, or specific vegetables to meet individual requirements, performance-enhancing salads offer flexibility while still maintaining their nutritional value.

Second, these salads promote proper hydration. Many vegetables and fruits used in performance-enhancing salads have high water content, which aids in hydration and helps athletes maintain optimal fluid balance during training and competitions. Proper hydration is essential for maintaining performance, preventing fatigue, and supporting recovery.

Performance-enhancing salads are a game-changer for athletes looking to optimize their nutrition and gain a competitive edge. These salads offer a nutrient-dense, well-balanced, and customizable meal option that supports energy, muscle recovery, hydration, and weight management. By incorporating performance-enhancing salads into their diets, athletes can nourish their bodies with a wide range of essential nutrients, enhance their physical performance, and achieve their athletic goals. As the understanding of the impact of nutrition on athletic performance continues to evolve, the role of performance-enhancing salads is set to become increasingly recognized and embraced by athletes at all levels.

QUINOA AND ROASTED VEGETABLE SALAD

Quinoa and Roasted Vegetable Salad is a nutritious and satisfying dish specifically designed to meet the dietary needs of athletes. This salad brings together the power of quinoa, a protein-rich grain, and an assortment of roasted vegetables to create a flavor-packed meal that supports athletic performance and recovery.

At the heart of this salad is quinoa, a complete protein that contains all nine essential amino acids necessary for muscle repair and growth. This grain is an excellent source of plant-based protein, making it an ideal choice for athletes following vegetarian or vegan diets. The protein content in quinoa helps to support muscle recovery after intense training sessions and promotes the development of lean muscle mass.

Complementing the quinoa are an array of roasted vegetables. These vegetables, such as bell peppers, zucchini, eggplant, and cherry tomatoes, are rich in essential vitamins, minerals, and antioxidants. The roasting process intensifies the flavors of the vegetables and brings out their natural sweetness. These nutrient-dense vegetables provide an abundance of vitamins A, C, and E, which are vital for immune function, reducing inflammation, and protecting the body against oxidative stress.

To further enhance the flavor profile and nutritional value, additional ingredients such as fresh herbs, lemon juice, and a drizzle of olive oil are added to the salad. Fresh herbs like basil, parsley, or cilantro not only add a burst of freshness but also contribute to the overall antioxidant and anti-inflammatory properties of the dish. Lemon juice provides a tangy brightness while also providing vitamin C, which aids in collagen synthesis and iron absorption. Olive oil, a heart-healthy fat, delivers a dose of monounsaturated fats that promote satiety, support hormone production, and reduce inflammation.

The combination of quinoa, roasted vegetables, and flavorful additions creates a well-rounded meal that provides athletes with a balance of carbohydrates, proteins, healthy fats, vitamins, minerals, and antioxidants. This combination supports sustained energy levels, muscle repair, immune function, and overall well-being. The fiber content in this salad promotes digestive health and helps athletes feel satisfied for longer periods, making it an excellent choice for weight management goals.

Overall, the Quinoa and Roasted Vegetable Salad is a delicious, versatile, and nutrient-packed option for athletes looking to fuel their bodies with wholesome ingredients. It offers a medley of flavors, textures, and essential nutrients that support optimal athletic performance, recovery, and overall health. Whether enjoyed as a post-workout meal, a light lunch, or a hearty dinner, this salad is sure to satisfy athletes' taste buds while nourishing their bodies.

Quinoa and Roasted Vegetable Salad offers numerous benefits to athletes. Firstly, the high protein content in quinoa supports muscle recovery and growth, essential for athletes looking to optimize their performance. As a complete protein, quinoa provides all nine essential amino acids, making it an ideal choice for athletes following plant-based diets.

Additionally, the combination of quinoa and roasted vegetables provides a wealth of vitamins, minerals, and antioxidants. These nutrients are essential for immune function, reducing inflammation, and protecting the body from oxidative stress, all of which are crucial for athletes' overall health and well-being.

Furthermore, the fiber-rich nature of quinoa and the assortment of roasted vegetables promote digestive health and provide a feeling of satiety. This helps athletes manage their weight and sustain energy levels throughout their training and competitions.

The Quinoa and Roasted Vegetable Salad also offers a versatile and customizable option for athletes. They can easily tailor the salad by adding or substituting vegetables, herbs, or dressings to meet their individual preferences and nutritional needs. This flexibility ensures that athletes can enjoy a nourishing and flavorful meal that supports their specific dietary requirements.

The Quinoa and Roasted Vegetable Salad provides athletes with a protein-packed, nutrient-dense, and customizable meal option. It supports muscle recovery, immune function, digestive health, and weight management, all of which are crucial for optimizing athletic performance. By incorporating this salad into their diet, athletes can enjoy a delicious and wholesome meal that fuels their bodies and helps them reach their athletic goals.

SESAME GINGER CHICKEN SALAD

Sesame Ginger Chicken Salad is a flavorful and nutritious dish designed to meet the specific dietary needs of athletes. This salad brings together the bold flavors of sesame and ginger with lean chicken breast and a medley of fresh vegetables, creating a delicious and energizing meal that supports athletic performance and recovery.

At the heart of this salad is lean chicken breast, a rich source of high-quality protein. Protein is essential for muscle repair, growth, and recovery, making it a crucial component of an athlete's diet. The chicken breast provides a lean source of protein that is low in fat, allowing athletes to meet their protein needs without excessive calorie intake.

The sesame ginger dressing adds a vibrant flavor profile to the salad. Sesame oil, a key ingredient, delivers a distinctive nutty taste while providing heart-healthy fats. Ginger, known for its anti-inflammatory properties, adds a refreshing kick and aids in digestion. Together, these ingredients create a tangy and aromatic dressing that enhances the overall taste of the salad.

Complementing the chicken and dressing are an assortment of fresh vegetables. Crisp lettuce, vibrant bell peppers, crunchy carrots, and zesty scallions offer a variety of textures and colors. These vegetables are packed with essential vitamins, minerals, and antioxidants that support immune function, reduce inflammation, and promote overall health. The fiber content in the vegetables promotes satiety, aids in digestion, and supports healthy weight management.

To add an extra crunch and boost of nutrients, the salad can be topped with sesame seeds or chopped nuts. Sesame seeds provide a source of healthy fats, minerals like calcium and magnesium, and antioxidants. Nuts, such as almonds or cashews, offer protein, healthy fats, and additional vitamins and minerals.

The Sesame Ginger Chicken Salad offers a delicious and nutrient-dense option for athletes. It provides high-quality protein, healthy fats, essential vitamins and minerals, and anti-inflammatory properties. By incorporating this salad into their diet, athletes can nourish their bodies, enhance muscle recovery, support immune function, and optimize their athletic performance.

SPINACH AND STRAWBERRY SALAD WITH PECANS

The Spinach and Strawberry Salad with Pecans is a delightful and nutritious dish tailored specifically for athletes. This salad combines the vibrant flavors of fresh spinach leaves, sweet strawberries, and crunchy pecans to create a well-rounded meal that supports athletic performance and overall well-being.

At the core of this salad is spinach, a leafy green vegetable that boasts an impressive array of nutrients. Spinach is rich in vitamins A, C, and K, as well as iron, calcium, and folate. These nutrients are essential for maintaining strong bones, supporting immune function, and promoting optimal oxygen transport to muscles. Additionally, spinach contains nitrates, which have been shown to enhance exercise performance and improve cardiovascular health.

The addition of strawberries adds a burst of sweetness and provides an excellent source of vitamin C and antioxidants. Vitamin C plays a crucial role in collagen synthesis, which supports joint health and aids in injury prevention for athletes. Antioxidants help combat oxidative stress caused by intense physical activity, reducing inflammation and promoting faster recovery.

To further enhance the flavor and nutritional profile, this salad incorporates pecans. Pecans are a nutrient-dense nut that offers a healthy dose of monounsaturated fats, fiber, and various vitamins and minerals. These healthy fats provide sustained energy, support hormone production, and contribute to heart health. The fiber content promotes digestive health, aids in weight management, and helps athletes feel satisfied after their meal.

CHICKPEA SALAD WITH LEMON TAHINI DRESSING

One such meal that perfectly combines taste and nutrition for athletes is the Chickpea Salad with Lemon Tahini Dressing. Packed with protein, fiber, and a burst of refreshing flavors, this salad is a winner for athletes looking to nourish their bodies.

The star ingredient of this salad is the humble chickpea, which is a nutritional powerhouse. Rich in plant-based protein, chickpeas aid in muscle repair and recovery after intense workouts. They are also an excellent source of dietary fiber, which promotes healthy digestion and helps maintain stable blood sugar levels, crucial for sustained energy throughout training sessions.

The lemon tahini dressing adds a tangy and creamy element to the salad, enhancing its taste and nutritional profile. Tahini, a paste made from sesame seeds, is packed with healthy fats and essential minerals like calcium and iron. The addition of lemon juice provides a refreshing burst of vitamin C, known for its antioxidant properties that help combat exercise-induced oxidative stress.

Accompanying the chickpeas and dressing are an array of colorful vegetables, such as crisp cucumber, juicy cherry tomatoes, and vibrant bell peppers. These vegetables are rich in vitamins, minerals, and antioxidants that support overall health and aid in post-exercise recovery. The salad is topped with a sprinkle of fresh herbs like parsley or cilantro, adding a touch of brightness and flavor.

Not only does this Chickpea Salad with Lemon Tahini Dressing provide a balanced combination of macronutrients, but it also satisfies taste buds, making it a go-to meal for athletes seeking a nutritious and delicious option. Whether enjoyed as a pre-workout fuel or a post-training recovery meal, this salad is sure to provide the nourishment athletes need to perform at their best.

The Chickpea Salad with Lemon Tahini Dressing offers numerous benefits for athletes, making it an ideal addition to their diet. Firstly, the salad is rich in protein, thanks to the chickpeas and tahini dressing. Protein is essential for muscle repair and growth, aiding in post-workout recovery and enhancing athletic performance.

Additionally, the high fiber content in chickpeas promotes healthy digestion and helps athletes feel satiated for longer periods, preventing overeating and aiding in weight management. The salad's colorful assortment of vegetables provides a range of vitamins, minerals, and antioxidants, supporting overall health and strengthening the immune system.

The lemon tahini dressing adds a burst of flavor while

providing healthy fats, calcium, and iron. These nutrients are crucial for maintaining energy levels and supporting optimal bodily functions during intense physical activity. The combination of these ingredients also helps stabilize blood sugar levels, ensuring a steady release of energy during workouts.

CHAPTER 4

FILLING AND FLAVORFUL LUNCHES

When it comes to fueling the body for athletic performance, the importance of a well-rounded and nutritious diet cannot be overstated. Athletes require meals that provide them with the energy, nutrients, and sustenance needed to support their active lifestyle and enhance their performance. One key aspect of a successful athlete's diet is a filling and flavorful lunch that satisfies their hunger while delivering a powerhouse of nutrients.

Lunchtime is a critical opportunity for athletes to refuel their bodies, replenish energy stores, and prepare for the second half of their day, whether it includes training, practice, or competition. A well-planned lunch can offer a myriad of benefits, including sustained energy, enhanced recovery, improved focus, and overall well-being.

Filling lunches should incorporate a balanced combination of macronutrients, including complex carbohydrates, lean proteins, and healthy fats. Complex carbohydrates, such as whole grains, quinoa, or sweet potatoes, provide a steady release of energy, ensuring athletes have the fuel they need to power through their activities.

Lean proteins, such as chicken breast, fish, tofu, or legumes, are essential for muscle repair and growth. These protein sources provide the necessary amino acids required to recover from intense workouts, aiding in the development of lean muscle mass and supporting overall athletic performance.

Including healthy fats in an athlete's lunch is equally important. Foods like avocados, nuts, seeds, and olive oil provide essential fatty acids, which play a crucial role in hormone production, joint health, and overall cellular function. Healthy fats also contribute to satiety, keeping athletes feeling fuller for longer and preventing unnecessary snacking or overeating.

Apart from macronutrients, athletes should also focus on incorporating an array of micronutrients into their lunch. This can be achieved by including a variety of colorful fruits and vegetables. These vibrant ingredients are rich in vitamins, minerals, and antioxidants that support the immune system, aid in recovery, and help combat exercise-induced oxidative stress.

Furthermore, athletes can enhance the flavor and nutritional profile of their lunches by incorporating herbs, spices, and healthy dressings. Herbs and spices not only add depth and complexity to meals but also provide additional antioxidants and anti-inflammatory properties. Dressings made with ingredients like lemon juice, vinegar, or Greek yogurt can add tanginess while offering beneficial nutrients.

Meal preparation plays a crucial role in ensuring athletes have access to filling and flavorful lunches throughout their busy schedules. By dedicating time to plan and prepare meals in advance, athletes can avoid relying on processed or unhealthy options and have complete control over the ingredients and portion sizes of their lunches.

Filling and flavorful lunches are a vital component of an athlete's diet. These meals provide the necessary energy, macronutrients, micronutrients, and flavor to support athletic performance, aid in recovery, and promote overall well-being. By incorporating a balanced combination of complex carbohydrates, lean proteins, healthy fats, and a variety of fruits and vegetables, athletes can fuel their bodies optimally and achieve their performance goals. With careful meal planning and preparation, athletes can ensure they have access to nutritious and delicious lunches that satisfy their hunger and set them up for success on and off the field or court.

GRILLED CHICKEN AND SWEET POTATO WRAPS

For athletes seeking a nutritious and convenient meal option, Grilled Chicken and Sweet Potato Wraps are a perfect choice. Packed with lean protein, complex carbohydrates, and a medley of flavorful ingredients, these wraps provide the necessary fuel and sustenance to support athletic performance.

The star of these wraps is the grilled chicken breast, which is not only a lean source of protein but also a rich source of essential amino acids. Protein is crucial for muscle repair, growth, and recovery, helping athletes maintain and develop their muscle mass.

Complementing the chicken is the inclusion of sweet potatoes. These nutrient-dense tubers provide complex carbohydrates that offer a sustained release of energy, supporting endurance and preventing mid-day energy crashes. Sweet potatoes are also rich in vitamins, minerals, and fiber, contributing to overall health and aiding in digestion.

The wraps are further enhanced with an array of colorful vegetables such as crisp lettuce, juicy tomatoes, and crunchy bell peppers. These vegetables not only add vibrant flavors and textures but also provide a variety of vitamins, minerals, and antioxidants, which support immune function and help combat exercise-induced inflammation.

To add a burst of flavor, the wraps can be drizzled with a tangy and creamy sauce, such as a Greek yogurt-based dressing or a zesty salsa. These sauces not only enhance the taste but also offer additional protein, calcium, and beneficial probiotics.

One of the greatest advantages of these wraps is their convenience. Athletes can prepare them in advance and enjoy them on the go. This makes them an ideal option for busy training days or when athletes are on the move and need a portable and satisfying meal.

Whether enjoyed as a post-workout recovery meal or as a nourishing lunch, Grilled Chicken and Sweet Potato Wraps provide athletes with a balanced combination of protein, complex carbohydrates, and essential nutrients. These wraps offer a delicious and convenient way to refuel, satisfy hunger, and support athletic performance.

Grilled Chicken and Sweet Potato Wraps offer numerous benefits for athletes, making them an excellent choice for their dietary needs. Firstly, the wraps provide a balanced combination of lean protein from grilled chicken and complex carbohydrates from sweet potatoes. This combination supports muscle repair, growth, and sustained energy levels for optimal athletic performance.

The inclusion of colorful vegetables adds essential vitamins, minerals, and antioxidants that support immune function, aid in recovery, and combat exercise-induced inflammation. Additionally, the wraps are a convenient and portable option for athletes, allowing them to enjoy a nutritious meal on the go, whether it's during training sessions or when traveling.

Preparing these wraps is relatively simple and can be done in advance for added convenience. Grilled chicken can be seasoned with herbs and spices and cooked ahead of time. Sweet potatoes can be baked or roasted until tender and sliced into strips. The wraps can be assembled by layering the grilled chicken, sweet potato strips, fresh vegetables, and optional sauces or dressings onto a whole grain tortilla. They can be rolled up tightly and secured with toothpicks or wrapped in foil for easy transport.

The wraps can be stored in the refrigerator and enjoyed throughout the week. This allows athletes to have a ready-to-eat meal that meets their nutritional needs whenever they need a quick and satisfying option.

WHOLE GRAIN TURKEY AND AVOCADO SANDWICHES

When it comes to nourishing the body and satisfying hunger, Whole Grain Turkey and Avocado Sandwiches are an excellent choice for athletes. These sandwiches offer a combination of high-quality protein, healthy fats, and complex carbohydrates, making them a well-rounded and nutritious option for fueling athletic performance.

The star of these sandwiches is the lean turkey breast, which provides a generous amount of protein. Protein is essential for athletes as it aids in muscle repair, growth, and recovery. It helps support the development of lean muscle mass, which is crucial for strength, power, and overall athletic performance.

Accompanying the turkey is the creamy and nutritious avocado. Avocados are rich in heart-healthy monounsaturated fats, which provide a source of sustained energy and promote satiety. These healthy fats also aid in nutrient absorption, support brain function, and contribute to overall cellular health.

The sandwiches offer complex carbohydrates. These carbohydrates provide a steady release of energy, supporting sustained performance during training or competition. Whole grain bread is also a good source of fiber, which aids in digestion and helps athletes feel fuller for longer periods, preventing unnecessary snacking or overeating.

To enhance the flavor and nutritional profile of the sandwiches, additional ingredients can be included. Fresh vegetables like crisp lettuce, juicy tomatoes, and crunchy bell peppers add texture, flavor, and a host of vitamins, minerals, and antioxidants. These nutrients support overall health, aid in recovery, and contribute to a strong immune system.

A light spread, such as mustard or Greek yogurt-based

dressing, can be added to provide tanginess and moisture without adding excessive calories or unhealthy fats. These spreads can also provide additional protein and beneficial probiotics.

The benefits of Whole Grain Turkey and Avocado Sandwiches extend beyond their nutrient composition. These sandwiches are easy to prepare and highly versatile. Athletes can customize their sandwiches with their favorite vegetables, spreads, or condiments to suit their taste preferences. They can also be made in advance, making them a convenient option for busy training days or when athletes are on the go.

Preparing these sandwiches is straightforward. Start by selecting high-quality whole grain bread that is rich in fiber and nutrients. Layer the slices with thinly sliced turkey breast, ripe avocado slices, and a generous amount of fresh vegetables. Add a spread or dressing of choice for added flavor and moisture. Top it off with the second slice of bread, press gently, and cut the sandwich into halves or quarters for easy handling.

These sandwiches can be enjoyed immediately or wrapped tightly in parchment paper or foil for later consumption. They can be stored in the refrigerator, making them a practical option for pre or post-workout meals, as well as for a quick and nutritious lunch.

BLACK BEAN AND QUINOA-STUFFED PEPPERS

Black Bean and Quinoa-Stuffed Peppers are a nutritious and flavorful meal that is perfect for athletes looking to fuel their bodies with a balanced combination of protein, complex carbohydrates, and essential nutrients. These stuffed peppers offer a variety of benefits and can be easily prepared as part of a well-rounded athlete's diet.

The star ingredients of this dish are black beans and quinoa. Black beans are a fantastic source of plant-based protein, offering athletes the necessary amino acids for muscle repair and growth. They are also rich in dietary fiber, which aids in digestion and helps maintain stable blood sugar levels, ensuring sustained energy throughout training sessions. Quinoa, on the other hand, is a gluten-free grain that provides complex carbohydrates. It supplies athletes with a slow-release source of energy, enhancing endurance and supporting optimal performance.

In addition to black beans and quinoa, the peppers themselves are packed with vitamins and minerals. Bell peppers, especially the brightly colored varieties, are rich in vitamin C, which is known for its immune-boosting properties and its role in collagen production, aiding in joint health and recovery. They also contain vitamin A, potassium, and folate, contributing to overall health and well-being.

Preparing these stuffed peppers is relatively straightforward. Begin by cutting the tops off the peppers and removing the seeds and membranes. Then, the peppers can be blanched in boiling water or baked in the oven to soften them. While the peppers are cooking, the black bean and quinoa filling can be prepared. The filling can include cooked quinoa, black beans, diced vegetables like onions and tomatoes, and an array of flavorful herbs and spices. This combination provides a delicious and nutritious stuffing for the peppers.

Once the filling is ready, it can be spooned into the cooked peppers, and the dish can be baked until the peppers are tender and the filling is heated through. This can be a great make-ahead option, as the stuffed peppers can be prepared in advance and reheated when needed.

The benefits of Black Bean and Quinoa-Stuffed Peppers for athletes are plentiful. Firstly, the high protein content from the black beans and quinoa aids in muscle repair, recovery, and overall strength. Additionally, the complex carbohydrates from the quinoa offer athletes a sustained source of energy, supporting endurance during intense workouts or training sessions.

The fiber-rich black beans and quinoa contribute to healthy digestion and help athletes feel satiated for longer periods, preventing unnecessary snacking and aiding in weight management. The inclusion of colorful bell peppers ensures a variety of essential vitamins, minerals, and antioxidants, supporting overall health and immune function.

Furthermore, the versatility of this dish allows athletes to customize it to their liking. They can incorporate additional vegetables, herbs, and spices to enhance the flavor and nutritional profile. The stuffed peppers can also be served with a side of fresh salad or paired with a lean protein source such as grilled chicken or tofu for a complete and balanced meal.

Black Bean and Quinoa-Stuffed Peppers provide athletes with a nourishing and satisfying meal option. This dish offers a combination of protein, complex carbohydrates, fiber, vitamins, and minerals that are essential for athletic performance, muscle recovery, and overall well-being. Whether enjoyed as a post-workout meal or a nutritious lunch, these stuffed peppers are a delicious and convenient

MEDITERRANEAN-STYLE TUNA SALAD

The Mediterranean-style Tuna Salad is a perfect option for athletes looking for a nutritious, flavorful, and satisfying meal. Inspired by the vibrant flavors of the Mediterranean region, this salad combines high-quality protein, heart-healthy fats, and an abundance of colorful vegetables to provide athletes with a well-rounded and nourishing dish.

At the core of this salad is tuna, a lean and protein-packed fish. Tuna is an excellent source of essential amino acids that aid in muscle repair, growth, and recovery, making it an ideal choice for athletes seeking to support their athletic performance. Additionally, tuna is rich in omega-3 fatty acids, which promote cardiovascular health, reduce inflammation, and support brain function.

The Mediterranean-style twist comes from the addition of an array of vibrant vegetables such as juicy tomatoes, crisp cucumbers, tangy olives, and crunchy bell peppers. These vegetables not only add a variety of flavors and textures but are also packed with vitamins, minerals, and antioxidants. These nutrients contribute to overall health, support the immune system, and help combat oxidative stress induced by intense workouts.

To elevate the flavors and nutritional profile further, the salad is dressed with a light and tangy dressing made with olive oil, lemon juice, and herbs like oregano and basil. Olive oil, a staple in the Mediterranean diet, provides healthy monounsaturated fats that are beneficial for heart health and aid in nutrient absorption. Lemon juice adds a refreshing zest while providing vitamin C and antioxidants.

One of the major benefits of the Mediterranean-style Tuna Salad is its versatility and adaptability to individual preferences and dietary needs. Athletes can customize the salad by adding additional ingredients like feta cheese, red onions, or chickpeas for added flavor, texture, and nutritional value. The salad can also be served over a bed of nutrient-rich leafy greens such as spinach or arugula, further boosting its fiber and vitamin content.

In addition to its delicious flavors and nutritional benefits, this salad is relatively easy to prepare. It requires minimal cooking, making it a time-efficient option for athletes with busy schedules. The tuna can be quickly seared or grilled, and the vegetables can be chopped and prepared in advance. With the dressing ingredients mixed together, athletes can assemble the salad just before serving, ensuring maximum freshness and flavor.

The Mediterranean-style Tuna Salad offers numerous benefits for athletes. Its protein-rich tuna supports muscle recovery and growth, while the colorful vegetables provide essential nutrients for overall health and performance. The inclusion of heart-healthy fats from olive oil and omega-3 fatty acids from tuna contribute to cardiovascular health and aid in reducing inflammation.

Moreover, this salad is low in carbohydrates and can be easily modified to suit specific dietary needs, such as low-carb or keto diets. The balanced combination of proteins, fats, and vegetables helps promote satiety, preventing unnecessary snacking and aiding in weight management.

The Mediterranean-style Tuna Salad is a nutritious and flavorful option for athletes seeking a well-rounded and satisfying meal. Packed with lean protein, heart-healthy fats, and an abundance of colorful vegetables, this salad offers numerous benefits, including muscle recovery and growth, cardiovascular health support, reduced inflammation, and overall well-being. With its versatility and easy preparation, athletes can enjoy a delicious and nourishing salad that fuels their bodies and enhances their athletic performance.

GRILLED SALMON AND MIXED GREENS SALAD

The Grilled Salmon and Mixed Greens Salad is a culinary masterpiece that combines the richness of grilled salmon with the freshness of mixed greens. Packed with flavor, essential nutrients, and a variety of textures, this salad offers a delightful and nourishing experience for those seeking a healthy and satisfying meal.

At the heart of this salad is the grilled salmon, a fatty fish renowned for its omega-3 fatty acids. These healthy fats are known for their anti-inflammatory properties, which can help reduce muscle soreness and promote cardiovascular health. Salmon is also an excellent source of high-quality protein, providing essential amino acids necessary for muscle repair and growth, making it an ideal choice for athletes.

The mixed greens in the salad add a refreshing and crisp element. This blend of nutrient-dense leafy greens, such as spinach, arugula, and romaine lettuce, provides an array of vitamins, minerals, and dietary fiber. These greens contribute to overall health, support digestion, and provide antioxidants that combat oxidative stress caused by intense physical activity.

Accompanying the greens are an assortment of colorful vegetables, such as vibrant cherry tomatoes, sliced cucumbers, and thinly sliced red onions. These vegetables not only enhance the visual appeal of the salad but also offer additional vitamins, minerals, and antioxidants that support immune function and aid in post-exercise recovery.

To elevate the taste and nutritional profile, the salad can be topped with a sprinkling of nutrient-rich ingredients like toasted nuts, such as almonds or walnuts, and seeds like chia or pumpkin seeds. These additions provide healthy fats, protein, and additional vitamins and minerals, adding both texture and flavor to the salad.

The dressing for the Grilled Salmon and Mixed Greens Salad can be a light vinaigrette made with olive oil, lemon juice, Dijon mustard, and a touch of honey or a tangy yogurt-based dressing. These dressings not only enhance the flavors but also provide heart-healthy fats, antioxidants, and probiotics, contributing to overall well-being.

One of the benefits of this salad is its versatility. It can be enjoyed as a light and refreshing lunch or as a satisfying dinner. The combination of protein from the salmon, fiber from the greens, and healthy fats from the dressing provides a balanced meal that keeps you feeling satiated and energized.

Preparing the Grilled Salmon and Mixed Greens Salad is relatively simple. Start by grilling or baking the salmon until it reaches a tender and flaky texture. Meanwhile, thoroughly wash and dry the mixed greens and vegetables. Slice and prepare the vegetables according to personal preference. Toss the greens and vegetables together in a large bowl, adding the toasted nuts and seeds if desired. Once the salmon is cooked, flake it into bite-sized pieces and gently place it on top of the salad. Finish by drizzling the dressing of your choice and gently tossing everything together until well-coated.

The Grilled Salmon and Mixed Greens Salad is a nutritious delight that combines the health benefits of salmon, mixed greens, and an assortment of colorful vegetables. It offers a well-rounded meal that supports muscle recovery, provides essential nutrients, and contributes to overall well-being. Whether enjoyed as a light lunch or a fulfilling dinner, this salad is a perfect choice for those seeking a flavorful, nutritious, and satisfying meal.

CHAPTER 5

NUTRIENT-DENSE DINNERS

Athletes dedicate themselves to pushing their bodies to the limits, seeking peak performance and excellence in their chosen sport. To achieve their goals, athletes must prioritize their nutrition, and one key component of their diet is nutrient-dense dinners. These meals play a vital role in fueling performance, optimizing recovery, and nourishing overall well-being.

Nutrient-dense dinners for athletes are carefully crafted meals that provide a concentrated amount of essential macronutrients, micronutrients, and phytochemicals. These dinners are designed to offer a wide array of vitamins, minerals, antioxidants, and other vital compounds that support the body's functions and aid in the recovery process.

A nutrient-dense dinner for athletes typically includes a balance of macronutrients: complex carbohydrates, lean proteins, and healthy fats. Complex carbohydrates, such as whole grains, quinoa, or sweet potatoes, serve as the primary source of energy, providing the necessary fuel for athletic activities and supporting glycogen replenishment.

Lean proteins, including chicken breast, turkey, fish, tofu, or legumes, play a crucial role in muscle repair and growth.

These proteins supply the body with essential amino acids required for rebuilding damaged muscle tissue and promoting recovery after intense training sessions or competitions.

Healthy fats are an essential component of nutrient-dense dinners for athletes. Avocados, nuts, seeds, olive oil, and fatty fish like salmon offer omega-3 fatty acids, which aid in reducing inflammation, supporting joint health, and promoting overall cellular function. Incorporating healthy fats also aids in the absorption of fat-soluble vitamins and helps athletes feel satiated, preventing overeating and unnecessary snacking.

In addition to macronutrients, nutrient-dense dinners prioritize the inclusion of an abundance of colorful and nutrient-rich vegetables. Leafy greens, cruciferous vegetables, peppers, tomatoes, and other vibrant options provide a wide range of vitamins, minerals, antioxidants, and fiber. These vegetables support overall health, boost the immune system, aid in recovery, and provide necessary phytonutrients that protect against exercise-induced oxidative stress.

Preparing nutrient-dense dinners for athletes involves careful planning and strategic meal composition. Athletes can benefit from prepping ingredients in advance, such as roasting vegetables, cooking whole grains, and batch-cooking proteins, to ensure quick and convenient meal assembly during busy training schedules.

Furthermore, incorporating herbs, spices, and healthy dressings can enhance the flavor profile of nutrient-dense dinners. Fresh herbs like basil, cilantro, or mint add brightness and depth to meals, while citrus juices, vinegar, or Greek yogurt-based dressings provide tanginess without excessive calories. The addition of aromatic spices not only elevates taste but also provides numerous health benefits, including anti-inflammatory properties.

The benefits of consuming nutrient-dense dinners are vast for athletes. These meals supply the necessary nutrients to support muscle recovery, optimize athletic performance, and enhance overall well-being. By providing the body with a balanced blend of macronutrients and an abundance of micronutrients, nutrient-dense dinners contribute to glycogen replenishment, muscle repair, immune system support, improved sleep quality, and long-term health maintenance.

Nutrient-dense dinners are a fundamental component of an athlete's dietary regimen. These meals serve as a powerful tool in fueling performance, promoting recovery, and nourishing the body. By incorporating a wide variety of whole foods, lean proteins, complex carbohydrates, healthy fats, and vibrant vegetables, athletes can optimize their nutrition and unlock their full potential. With mindful meal planning, preparation, and a focus on nutrient density, athletes can enjoy delicious and satisfying dinners that propel them towards their athletic goals while supporting their overall health and well-being.

GRILLED LEMON PEPPER CHICKEN WITH ROASTED VEGETABLES

For athletes, a well-rounded and nutrient-dense meal is essential to fuel their performance and support their recovery. The combination of Grilled Lemon Pepper Chicken with Roasted Vegetables offers a delicious and wholesome option that satisfies hunger, provides an abundance of vital nutrients, and aids in athletic success.

At the center of this meal is the lean and protein-rich grilled chicken. Chicken breast is a staple for athletes as it contains all the essential amino acids necessary for muscle repair and growth. The lemon pepper seasoning adds a zesty and tangy flavor to the chicken, enhancing its taste while providing the added benefits of vitamin C and antioxidants from the lemon.

Accompanying the grilled chicken are a medley of roasted vegetables. Roasting vegetables like bell peppers, zucchini, carrots, and broccoli enhances their natural flavors and textures while preserving their valuable nutrients. These colorful vegetables are packed with vitamins, minerals, fiber, and antioxidants, which support overall health, aid in recovery, and combat exercise-induced oxidative stress.

TERIYAKI SALMON WITH BROWN RICE AND BOK CHOY

For athletes seeking a flavorful and nutrient-dense meal, Teriyaki Salmon with Brown Rice and Bok Choy is an excellent choice. This dish combines the richness of salmon, the wholesome goodness of brown rice, and the vibrant freshness of bok choy to create a meal that nourishes the body and supports athletic performance.

Salmon takes center stage in this dish as a lean source of protein and a rich source of omega-3 fatty acids. Protein is vital for muscle repair and growth, allowing athletes to recover effectively and build lean muscle mass. Omega-3 fatty acids provide numerous benefits, including reducing inflammation, supporting heart health, and promoting brain function. The combination of protein and healthy fats in salmon provides sustained energy and aids in post-workout recovery.

The teriyaki glaze adds a sweet and savory flavor to the salmon while providing an additional burst of taste. However, it's essential to choose a teriyaki sauce with minimal added sugars and artificial ingredients to maximize the health benefits of the dish.

Accompanying the salmon is brown rice, a whole grain rich

in fiber, vitamins, and minerals. Brown rice provides complex carbohydrates, supplying long-lasting energy and helping athletes sustain their performance. The fiber content aids in digestion, promotes satiety, and supports healthy blood sugar levels.

CHAPTER 6

RECOVERY SMOOTHIES AND SHAKES

As athletes push their bodies to the limit during intense training sessions and competitions, their nutritional needs become paramount for optimal performance and recovery. One key element in their nutrition regimen is the consumption of recovery smoothies and shakes. These delicious concoctions offer a convenient and effective way to replenish vital nutrients, support muscle repair, and promote overall recovery. In this introduction, we will explore the benefits, ingredients, and strategies behind recovery smoothies and shakes for athletes.

Athletes put tremendous stress on their bodies, leading to the depletion of essential nutrients, muscle damage, and the accumulation of metabolic waste products. Proper nutrition and efficient recovery play pivotal roles in maximizing athletic performance and reducing the risk of injuries. Recovery smoothies and shakes have gained popularity among athletes as they offer a quick and easily digestible solution to restore energy levels, aid in muscle repair, and promote the body's recovery process.

One of the primary benefits of recovery smoothies and shakes is their ability to deliver a concentrated dose of nutrients in a convenient and efficient manner. These beverages are often packed with high-quality proteins, carbohydrates, vitamins, minerals, and antioxidants—all essential for replenishing energy stores and supporting muscle recovery. By blending these ingredients into a liquid form, the nutrients are more easily absorbed by the body, allowing for faster delivery to the muscles and other tissues that need them the most.

Protein is a vital component of recovery smoothies and shakes for athletes. It plays a crucial role in muscle repair and growth, helping to rebuild damaged muscle fibers after strenuous exercise. Whey protein, derived from milk, is a popular choice due to its high biological value and fast absorption rate. Other sources of protein commonly used include plant-based options like pea, hemp, and brown rice protein, suitable for athletes following a vegetarian or vegan diet.

Carbohydrates are another essential ingredient in recovery beverages, as they replenish glycogen stores that become depleted during exercise. The optimal carbohydrate-to-protein ratio in these shakes varies depending on the athlete's specific needs and the type of exercise performed. For endurance athletes, a higher carbohydrate content may be beneficial, while those engaged in strength training might opt for a higher protein ratio. Adding fruits, such as bananas or berries, to the shakes provides not only a source of carbohydrates but also additional vitamins, minerals, and antioxidants.

In addition to protein and carbohydrates, recovery smoothies and shakes often incorporate healthy fats, such as nut butters, avocados, or flaxseed oil. These fats provide a source of long-lasting energy and help promote satiety, making the shakes more satisfying and sustaining for athletes. Including a small amount of fat also aids in the absorption of fat-soluble vitamins present in the other ingredients.

To enhance the recovery process further, many athletes choose to supplement their smoothies and shakes with additional ingredients known for their anti-inflammatory and antioxidant properties. Examples of such ingredients include turmeric, ginger, spinach, kale, or chia seeds. These powerful additions help combat exercise-induced inflammation, reduce muscle soreness, and support the body's overall recovery mechanisms.

Timing is crucial when it comes to consuming recovery smoothies and shakes. Athletes are encouraged to consume these beverages within the post-exercise "window of opportunity," which is typically 30 minutes to two hours after training or competition. During this timeframe, the body is primed to absorb and utilize nutrients most efficiently, maximizing the benefits of the recovery beverage.

Recovery smoothies and shakes are a valuable tool for athletes to replenish their bodies after intense physical activity. These nutrient-dense beverages provide the essential ingredients needed for efficient muscle repair, glycogen replenishment, and overall recovery. By incorporating protein, carbohydrates, healthy fats, and additional anti-inflammatory ingredients, athletes can optimize their post-workout nutrition and enhance their athletic performance. With their convenience and versatility, recovery smoothies and shakes have become a favored choice among athletes striving for optimal recovery and sustained success.

BANANA AND ALMOND BUTTER PROTEIN SHAKE

The combination of bananas and almond butter in a protein shake has become a go-to choice for athletes looking to refuel and recover effectively after intense workouts. This delicious and nutritious shake provides a host of benefits that support muscle repair, replenish energy stores, and promote overall athletic performance. In this description, we will delve into the key ingredients, nutritional profile, and advantages of the Banana and Almond Butter Protein Shake for athletes.

The star ingredients of this protein shake are bananas and almond butter. Bananas are a fantastic source of natural carbohydrates, providing a quick and easily digestible energy source for athletes. They are rich in potassium, a mineral essential for maintaining proper muscle function and preventing cramping. Bananas also contain vitamins C and B6, as well as dietary fiber, promoting healthy digestion and overall well-being.

Almond butter, on the other hand, contributes healthy fats, protein, and a range of important nutrients to the shake. The inclusion of almond butter not only enhances the taste and creaminess of the shake but also provides a satiating effect that keeps athletes feeling full and satisfied. Almond butter is an excellent source of monounsaturated fats, which support heart health and provide a sustained source of energy. It also contains protein, which is crucial for muscle repair and growth.

In addition to bananas and almond butter, this protein shake typically includes a high-quality protein powder. Whey protein is a popular choice among athletes due to its complete amino acid profile and rapid absorption rate. However, plant-based protein powders, such as pea, soy, or hemp, are also viable options for athletes following vegetarian or vegan diets. The protein component of the shake plays a vital role in repairing damaged muscle tissue and promoting muscle growth, ensuring athletes recover optimally and adapt to their training regimen.

The Banana and Almond Butter Protein Shake offers numerous benefits to athletes. First and foremost, it delivers a balanced combination of macronutrients, including carbohydrates, protein, and healthy fats. This blend of nutrients is crucial for replenishing glycogen stores, supporting muscle recovery, and providing sustained energy for the body. The carbohydrates from the banana, combined with the protein from the almond butter and protein powder, create an ideal post-workout shake that jump-starts the recovery process.

Another advantage of this protein shake is its versatility and convenience. It can be easily prepared within minutes, making it a practical choice for busy athletes. The shake can be consumed immediately after a workout or as a quick meal replacement option for athletes on the go. It also serves as a healthier alternative to processed snacks or sugary drinks commonly consumed after exercise, supporting athletes in making nutritious choices that align with their fitness goals.

The Banana and Almond Butter Protein Shake offers a range of additional nutritional benefits. It contains essential vitamins and minerals, including potassium, magnesium, and vitamins C and B6, which support overall health and well-being. The shake also provides dietary fiber, aiding digestion and promoting a healthy gut.

The Banana and Almond Butter Protein Shake is a highly beneficial choice for athletes seeking a delicious and nutrient-packed post-workout beverage. With the natural carbohydrates from bananas, protein from almond butter and protein powder, and a range of essential vitamins and minerals, this shake delivers the necessary fuel and building blocks for muscle recovery and optimal athletic performance. Its convenience and versatility make it an excellent option for athletes looking to refuel efficiently and nourish their bodies effectively.

BERRY BLAST RECOVERY SMOOTHIE

The Berry Blast Recovery Smoothie is a delicious and nutrient-packed beverage designed specifically to aid athletes in their post-workout recovery. Bursting with the vibrant flavors of various berries, this smoothie combines an array of beneficial ingredients to replenish energy stores, support muscle repair, and promote overall recovery. Let's explore the description and key benefits of the Berry Blast Recovery Smoothie for athletes.

The Berry Blast Recovery Smoothie is made with a blend of antioxidant-rich berries, including strawberries, blueberries, and raspberries. These berries not only provide a burst of sweetness but also deliver a multitude of vitamins, minerals, and phytochemicals essential for optimal recovery. The vibrant colors of the berries are indicative of their high antioxidant content, which helps combat exercise-induced oxidative stress and inflammation, reducing the risk of muscle damage and enhancing recovery.

This recovery smoothie also contains a high-quality protein source, such as whey or plant-based protein powder, which supports muscle repair and growth. Protein is crucial for athletes as it aids in the synthesis of new muscle tissue and helps rebuild damaged muscle fibers after intense exercise. By incorporating protein into the Berry Blast Recovery Smoothie, athletes can provide their bodies with the necessary building blocks for efficient muscle recovery.

Carbohydrates play a vital role in replenishing glycogen stores that become depleted during exercise. The Berry Blast Recovery Smoothie includes a source of carbohydrates, typically in the form of fruits like bananas or mangoes, which not only provide natural sweetness but also supply the energy needed for recovery. The combination of carbohydrates and protein in this smoothie helps kickstart the recovery process by delivering essential nutrients to the muscles, restoring glycogen levels, and supporting tissue repair.

To enhance the nutritional profile of the Berry Blast Recovery Smoothie, healthy fats may be added, such as a tablespoon of almond butter or a drizzle of flaxseed oil. These fats not only provide a source of sustained energy but also aid in the absorption of fat-soluble vitamins present in the smoothie. Additionally, the smoothie may include additional ingredients like Greek yogurt, spinach, or chia seeds to further boost its nutritional content and provide added benefits such as probiotics, iron, and omega-3 fatty acids.

The benefits of the Berry Blast Recovery Smoothie are numerous. Firstly, it helps replenish energy stores, providing athletes with the fuel they need for their next training session or competition. Secondly, the high protein content supports muscle recovery and growth, reducing muscle soreness and enhancing overall performance. The antioxidant-rich berries combat inflammation and oxidative stress, promoting a faster recovery process and reducing the risk of injuries. Lastly, the inclusion of healthy fats and other nutrient-dense ingredients ensures a well-rounded and balanced nutritional profile, supporting overall health and well-being.

The Berry Blast Recovery Smoothie is a delicious and nutritious option for athletes seeking optimal post-workout recovery. Packed with antioxidant-rich berries, protein, carbohydrates, and healthy fats, this smoothie delivers a powerhouse of nutrients to support muscle repair, replenish energy stores, and reduce inflammation. By incorporating the Berry Blast Recovery Smoothie into their nutrition regimen, athletes can enhance their recovery process, improve performance, and maintain overall well-being.

CHOCOLATE AVOCADO PROTEIN SMOOTHIE

The Chocolate Avocado Protein Smoothie is a delicious and nutritious beverage specifically designed to support the recovery and performance of athletes. This smoothie combines the rich flavors of chocolate with the creamy goodness of avocado to create a delightful blend that not only satisfies the taste buds but also provides essential nutrients to fuel the body after intense exercise.

One of the key ingredients in this smoothie is avocado, which brings both creaminess and a host of health benefits. Avocados are an excellent source of healthy fats, including monounsaturated fats, which are known to support heart health and reduce inflammation. These fats contribute to the smoothie's satiety and provide long-lasting energy for athletes. Avocados also contain a wide range of vitamins and minerals, including potassium, vitamin K, vitamin E, and B vitamins, which help support overall health and wellbeing.

Another essential component of the Chocolate Avocado Protein Smoothie is the protein content. Protein is crucial for muscle repair and growth, making it an indispensable nutrient for athletes. In this smoothie, a high-quality protein powder, such as whey or plant-based protein, is added to ensure an adequate intake of this macronutrient. Protein helps to repair damaged muscle tissue, supports the development of lean muscle mass, and aids in the overall recovery process after intense workouts or competitions.

The addition of chocolate to this smoothie not only enhances its flavor but also offers some surprising benefits. Dark chocolate, in particular, contains flavonoids and antioxidants, which have been associated with improved cardiovascular health, enhanced cognitive function, and reduced inflammation. It can also provide a natural mood boost, making the post-workout recovery period more enjoyable.

GREEN POWER SMOOTHIE WITH SPINACH AND KALE

The Green Power Smoothie with Spinach and Kale is a nutrient-packed beverage that has gained popularity among athletes for its numerous benefits in supporting performance and recovery. This vibrant green smoothie is made with a blend of spinach, kale, and other ingredients that provide a potent dose of essential vitamins, minerals, antioxidants, and phytochemicals.

This smoothie is an excellent choice for athletes looking to increase their intake of leafy greens, as spinach and kale are known for their high nutrient content. Spinach is rich in iron, which plays a crucial role in oxygen transport and energy production. It also provides an abundance of vitamins A, C, and K, along with folate and magnesium. Kale, on the other hand, is packed with antioxidants, fiber, and vitamins C and K, promoting healthy digestion, immune function, and bone health.

The Green Power Smoothie also incorporates other ingredients to enhance its nutritional profile. A typical recipe might include a source of high-quality protein such as Greek yogurt or a plant-based protein powder. Protein is essential for muscle repair and growth, making it an integral component of post-workout recovery for athletes. Additionally, the smoothie might include fruits like bananas or berries, which contribute natural sugars and additional vitamins and minerals to support energy replenishment and overall health.

One of the main benefits of this smoothie for athletes is its ability to aid in post-exercise recovery. The combination of leafy greens, protein, and carbohydrates helps replenish glycogen stores, repair muscle tissue, and reduce exercise-induced inflammation. The antioxidants found in spinach and kale assist in combating oxidative stress caused by intense physical activity, supporting the body's recovery processes and reducing muscle soreness.

The Green Power Smoothie provides a convenient and efficient way for athletes to meet their daily nutritional needs. It can be easily prepared in advance and consumed on the go, making it an ideal option for busy athletes. By incorporating this smoothie into their post-workout routine, athletes can ensure they are fueling their bodies with the essential nutrients needed for optimal performance and recovery.

TROPICAL PINEAPPLE AND COCONUT POST-WORKOUT SHAKE

The Tropical Pineapple and Coconut Post-Workout Shake is a refreshing and nutritious beverage designed specifically for athletes to support their recovery after intense physical activity. This delicious shake combines the tropical flavors of pineapple and coconut with key ingredients that aid in muscle repair, replenish energy stores, and promote overall recovery.

The shake begins with a base of coconut water, which serves as a natural electrolyte-rich fluid to rehydrate the body after exercise. Coconut water is not only hydrating but also provides essential minerals like potassium, magnesium, and sodium, which are crucial for restoring electrolyte balance and preventing muscle cramps.

The star ingredient, pineapple, offers a burst of tropical sweetness while providing numerous benefits for athletes. Pineapple contains bromelain, a natural enzyme known for its anti-inflammatory properties. By reducing inflammation, bromelain helps alleviate muscle soreness and promotes faster recovery. Pineapple is also rich in vitamin C, an antioxidant that supports the immune system and aids in collagen synthesis, crucial for maintaining healthy connective tissues.

To enhance the nutritional profile, a high-quality protein source is added to the shake. Whey protein is commonly used due to its fast absorption rate and complete amino acid profile, which supports muscle repair and growth. Alternatively, plant-based proteins like pea or brown rice can be used for athletes following a vegetarian or vegan diet.

The shake is rounded out with a dose of healthy fats from coconut milk or coconut oil. These fats provide sustained energy, enhance satiety, and facilitate the absorption of fat-soluble vitamins. They also add a creamy texture and tropical flavor to the shake.

By consuming the Tropical Pineapple and Coconut Post-Workout Shake, athletes can enjoy several benefits. Firstly, the high-quality protein aids in muscle repair, reducing the risk of muscle breakdown and promoting growth. Secondly, the carbohydrates from pineapple and coconut water replenish glycogen stores, restoring energy levels for optimal performance in subsequent workouts or competitions. Additionally, the anti-inflammatory properties of pineapple help reduce exercise-induced inflammation, minimizing muscle soreness and enhancing overall recovery.

The convenience of this shake makes it an ideal option for

busy athletes who require a quick and easily digestible post-workout meal. Its portable nature allows athletes to consume it immediately after exercise, taking advantage of the crucial post-exercise "window of opportunity" when nutrient absorption is optimal.

The Tropical Pineapple and Coconut Post-Workout Shake offers a delicious and nutrient-packed option for athletes looking to maximize their recovery. With its blend of pineapple, coconut water, protein, and healthy fats, this shake provides hydration, essential nutrients, and anti-inflammatory properties—all crucial for efficient muscle repair, glycogen replenishment, and overall recovery. By incorporating this shake into their post-workout routine, athletes can optimize their nutrition, enhance their athletic performance, and stay on top of their game.

CHAPTER 7

MEAL PLANS

Here's a sample day-by-day meal plan for an athlete:

Day 1:

Breakfast: Veggie omelet with spinach, mushrooms, and bell peppers. Whole-grain toast with avocado.

Snack: Greek yogurt with mixed berries and a sprinkle of nuts.

Lunch: Grilled chicken breast with quinoa and roasted vegetables.

Snack: Apple slices with almond butter.

Dinner: Baked salmon with steamed asparagus and brown rice.

Post-workout Snack: Protein shake with banana and almond milk.

Day 2:

Breakfast: High fiber granola bars

Snack: Protein bar and a handful of almonds.

Lunch: Turkey wrap with whole-grain tortilla, lean turkey, mixed greens, and hummus.

Snack: Carrot sticks with hummus.

Dinner: Lean beef stir-fry with broccoli, bell peppers, and brown rice.

Post-workout Snack: Chocolate milk or a protein smoothie.

Day 3:

Breakfast: Whole-grain pancakes topped with Greek yogurt and berries.

Snack: Homemade trail mix with dried fruits and nuts.

Lunch: Quinoa salad with mixed greens, grilled chicken, cherry tomatoes, and avocado.

Snack: Cottage cheese with pineapple chunks.

Dinner: Grilled shrimp with quinoa pilaf and roasted vegetables.

Post-workout Snack: Peanut butter and banana smoothie.

Day 4:

Breakfast: Scrambled eggs with spinach, tomatoes, and whole-grain toast.

Snack: Rice cakes with almond butter.

Lunch: Grilled tofu with brown rice noodles and stir-fried vegetables.

Snack: Greek yogurt with honey and sliced almonds.

Dinner: Baked chicken breast with sweet potato wedges and steamed broccoli.

Post-workout Snack: Protein bar and a piece of fruit.

Day 5:

Breakfast: Spinach and feta cheese omelet with whole-grain toast.

Snack: Homemade protein balls.

Lunch: Quinoa-stuffed bell peppers with a side salad.

Snack: Sliced cucumbers with hummus.

Dinner: Grilled salmon with quinoa and roasted Brussels sprouts.

Post-workout Snack: Mixed berry smoothie with protein powder.

Remember to adjust portion sizes and caloric intake based on individual needs and training intensity. It's also essential to stay hydrated throughout the day by drinking plenty of water.

Conclusion:

In conclusion, "The Athlete's Cookbook" provides a comprehensive guide to nourishing the body and optimizing performance through delicious and nutritious meals. This book has taken readers on a culinary journey, exploring the intersection of taste, fitness, and overall well-being. By presenting a wide range of recipes tailored specifically to athletes, it empowers individuals to fuel their bodies efficiently, enhance recovery, and achieve their full potential. Beyond the kitchen, it emphasizes the importance of mindful eating, emphasizing the relationship between food and athletic success. With its practical tips, flavorful recipes, and insightful advice, "The Athlete's Cookbook" has become an indispensable resource for athletes of all levels, inspiring them to excel both on and off the field.